Virgin Diet Review

Lose Weight, intelligently

I0435679

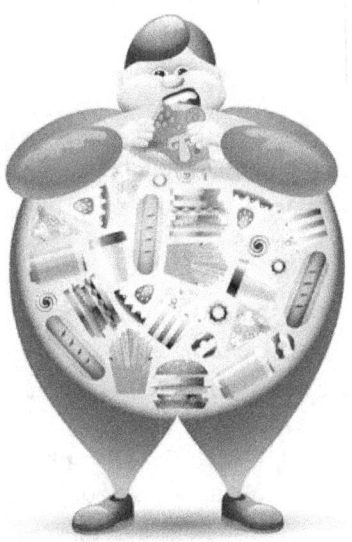

Health Learning Series

M. Usman

Mendon Cottage Books

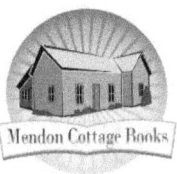

JD-Biz Publishing

Disclaimer

The information is this book is provided for informational purposes only. It is not intended to be used and medical advice or a substitute for proper medical treatment by a qualified health care provider. The information is believed to be accurate as presented based on research by the author.

The contents have not been evaluated by the U.S. Food and Drug Administration or any other Government or Health Organization and the contents in this book are not to be used to treat cure or prevent disease.

The author or publisher is not responsible for the use or safety of any diet, procedure or treatment mentioned in this book. The author or publisher is not responsible for errors or omissions that may exist.

Warning

The Book is for informational purposes only and before taking on any diet, treatment or medical procedure, it is recommended to consult with your primary health care provider.

Our books are available at

1. Amazon.com
2. Barnes and Noble
3. Itunes
4. Kobo
5. Smashwords
6. Google Play Books

Table of Contents

Prelude

The Virgin Diet was created by J.J. Virgin, a nutritionist and celebrity fitness expert since 1987. JJ was the author of the extremely popular book, "The Virgin Diet", which is the basis for this book. If it wasn't for her, this book might never have gotten into the pipeline.

The weight-loss industry has become a multi-billion dollar venture with enterprises, medical field-experts, and nutritionists struggling to get the biggest slice of the profits. In this race for fame and fortune, some people actually work to make a product that would last a long time while many produce a one-time thing that will waste the consumer's money and health. The "Virgin Diet" is the former of the two cases. It is a tried and tested diet that will shave off extra pounds from your body using a systematic approach. So before you move on to forthcoming chapters, you must be absolutely focused and sure that this diet will work, as mental awareness is as important as the physical one!

Assuming that you are new to this fitness-world; this book will get you nicely delved into the world of diets, especially "the Virgin Diet".

Don't over think, make up your mind and get ready to get those calories off of you!

Getting Started

Chapter 1: Overview

Before going ahead with the diet, let's discuss a little about the world of diets. You might have noticed that right before a holiday season, new diets start popping up in the market with excellent advertisement staff to lure you into the illusion of the biggest bang for your buck. I am not stating that all these diets are bad, but you should always carry out your own research before falling prey to these meaningless, so called, health wonders. These diets may offer something extra on the side or a medical secret to help you lose weight, but the reality of it is that they do nothing but take your money.

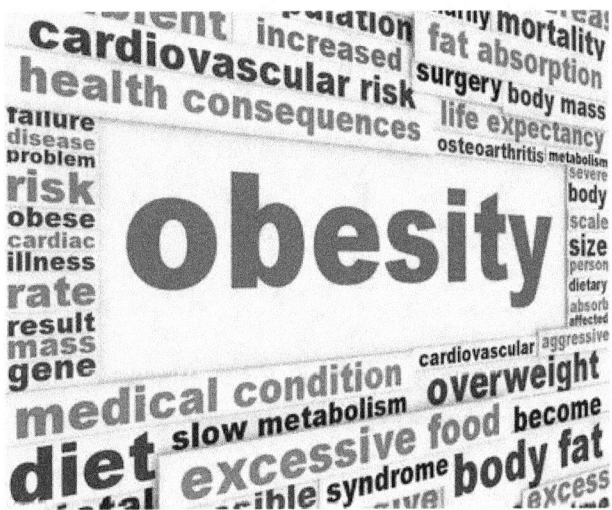

With the Virgin Diet, you will actually find scientific proof that will lead you to believe that it actually works. Getting right to the point, the Virgin Diet is a diet that will help you lose weight by the elimination of foods that cause you intolerance. The Virgin Diet proudly claims, "Lose 7 pounds in 7 days by dropping 7 foods".

An outline of the diet is as follows:

- Elimination of soy, eggs, dairy, corn, gluten, peanuts, sweeteners and sugars.

- Inclusion of whole, unprocessed natural foods that are locally raised.

- Consumption of Virgin Diet Shakes.

- Reintroduction and analysis of the reactions that stir up once eggs and dairy are again made a part of the diet; the time required to reintroduce these two classes of foods is found out.

- Reintroduction of soy and gluten to check the same thing as in the previous point.

- Avoidance of foods that cause trouble, other than those listed in the first point.

The science behind this diet is better explained in the next chapter. For now you need to cozy up with the diet book and open yourself to the idea of losing weight.

Chapter 2: Diving Deeper

As promised, the basis of this diet will be explained and you will not be led to believe that it somehow works, but there are a few misconceptions within the minds of the masses that need to be cleared first.

Over a third of the population believes that they are sufferers of food allergies. Research has categorically shown this statement to be false and stated that only 5% of the population actually does have allergies. Part of the problem for this behavior is the misuse and misunderstanding of the term "allergy" by people, which is quite different from food sensitivity and food intolerance. Here is a brief overview of all three terms:

- A **food allergy** is an immune response generated by the body to a specific food protein. The immune system responds to this protein by the production of an immunoglobin called IgE followed by release of histamine that causes hives, itching, dizziness, breathing problems or other symptoms.

- A **food intolerance,** on the other hand, is the absence of a food enzyme vital for food digestion. This is the reason behind gluten intolerance or lactose intolerance. Symptoms of food intolerance include constipation, diarrhea, GI upset, rashes or nasal congestion; the signs are normally not life-threatening.

- A **food sensitivity,** in turn, is an unpleasant reaction to a class of food items; the reaction includes symptoms like cramps, nausea, and heartburn and is usually not recurring after the same food is consumed.

So by now everything should have started to make much more sense and it should be clear that in order to remain perfectly healthy, you need to avoid foods that bring up any of the above reactions.

Mark Hyman, MD is the chairman of the Institute of Functional Medicine and he strongly believes that food allergies and sensitivities play an important role in the increase of one's body weight. Mr. Hyman made observations in hundreds of patients before setting out his claim, which has now been stamped by new research. Mr. Hyman stated that problems with the body's systems, like the immune system, gut and hormones, linked together to keep the body from not losing weight that was no good for it in the first place. A linkage was thus discovered between inflammation and weight loss and from there a basis for this diet was set out.

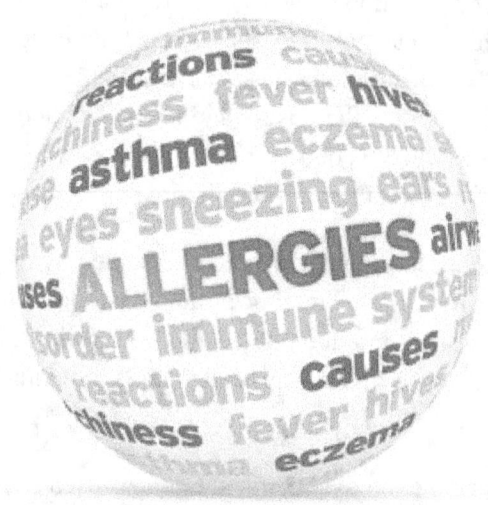

The first study that aimed to establish link between weight gain and inflammation was published in 2007. It looked at two collections of children; the first one being overweight with the second one being of normal weight. The scientists measured out three factors that were connected to inflammation to analyze their study.

- Firstly, they kept the C-reactive protein in check which is a well-established marker for inflammation in the body.

- Secondly, they looked for thickening of the carotid arteries with the deposit of plaque.

- Thirdly, they measured the percentage of IgGs that indicated food allergies.

The following discoveries were made:

- The obese kids had three-fold higher levels of the protein and two-and-a-half fold higher levels of IgG.

- The obese kids also had thicker arteries clogged with plaque which was an early indicator for heart disease and atherosclerosis.

The author of the study therefore showed that allergies were a cause of inflammation and not a consequence. He further reiterated his point by explaining that the damage to the gut results in a leaky gut, which allows the food particles to be exposed to the gut's internal immune system. This leads to a system-wide response from the immune system resulting in inflammation in all parts of body and resistance to weight loss by increasing resistance to insulin.

It is already known that inflammation from entities like bacteria, sugars and fats produce insulin resistance that leads to high levels of insulin. Since insulin helps store fat, the body gets resistive to weight loss mechanisms.

Another study was carried out that was aimed to find out how the gut leaked. The researchers selected a host of thin mice and fed them with a diet that was high in fats. The high fat diet changed the bacterial flora in the gut promoting the well-being of toxin producing bugs and reducing the number of bacteria that were entrusted with the role of fighting them. The researchers found out that when mice were fed with this diet, a bacterial toxin called LPS was produced which leaked through the gut wreaking havoc in the body.

Similarly, when we consume a low-fiber, high-sugar, highly processed diet along with antibiotics, it alters our guts' ecosystem and leads to inflammation. In humans, the toxins latch onto the immune cells and then cause a frenzy of inflammatory molecules which disturbs the body's metabolism.

When mice were injected with LPS, the same problems came up. Inflammation was followed by obesity. This proved that the toxins were at work and they did have a role in upsetting the natural balance of the body.

When you eat a fat-filled diet like the typical American Diet, the bad bacteria grow by leaps and folds and damage the lining of the gut, producing toxins that are then absorbed into the system. The partially digested food particles then leak into the bloodstream through holes in the gut's lining leading to a toxic liver and insulin resistant body; the ultimate result of which is obesity.

The Virgin Diet accomplished weight loss by this mechanism; it drops the foods that cause imbalances in the body and with that promote weight loss. The details of the foods are given in the next chapter.

Chapter 3: Foods to Drop

JJ Virgins, the developer of the Virgin Diet, carried out a detailed research before writing the book. She worked with top medical practitioners and doctors to find out the causes of obesity and came to the conclusion that it was elimination of a class of foods that brought relief and order to the body.

1.   **Gluten**:

Gluten plays a hand in triggering the release of the protein, zonulin that creates spaces between the junctions of the small intestine making it more permeable, allowing particles to move through it and creating an immune reaction attributed to inflammation.

2.   **Soy:**

Soy nowadays is heavily mutated, sprayed with pesticides and highly processed. It interferes with the thyroid's nominal functions and damages the gut.

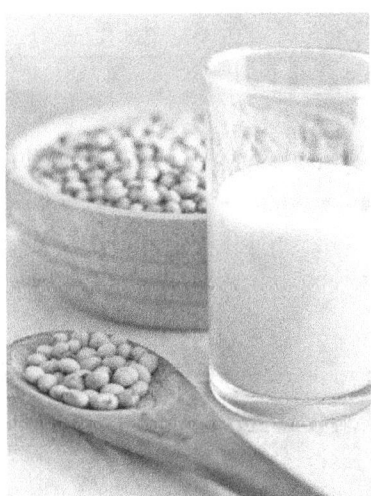

3.   **Eggs**:

Eggs are high in pro-inflammatory arachidonic acid that leads to various intolerances in the body.

4. **Dairy**:

Dairy just might be the most controversial food item on the list. Milk is high in lactose which is a sugar that heightens insulin resistance and causes imbalances in blood sugar. Studies have repeatedly shown that dairy can trigger acne and other conditions. Furthermore, the nurse's health study showed that those nurses with the highest consumption record for dairy had the highest occurrence of osteoporosis. Therefore consume seeds, nuts and leafy vegetables if you just want to build stronger bones.

5. **Peanuts**:

Peanuts are prone to molds and a fungus known as aflatoxin. Their fatty acid profile is not as healthy as other tree nuts and moreover all packed peanuts are relatively high in trans fats and corn syrup which is not at all beneficial for the body.

6. **Corn**:

Corn is high glycemic, inflammatory and on top of that genetically modified; no way that's going to do any good.

7. **Sugars**:

Sugar is already known for a host of problems. Artificial sweeteners are actually worse than natural sugar; their sweetness triggers an insulin response leading to gain in weight. A simple study showed that people who consumed diet-sodas gained more weight as compared to those who drank simple sodas.

You only need to remove these 7 foods for 3 weeks to benefit from the diet; 3 weeks is not that long a time and you can easily replace these foods with healthier combos! Get ready as it gets real from here on out.

The Cycles of Virgin Diet

Chapter 1: Elimination

This is the first stage of the Virgin Diet and it lasts for 3 weeks; all foods that cause imbalances in the system are cut out and healing foods are included in the diet as their replacements.

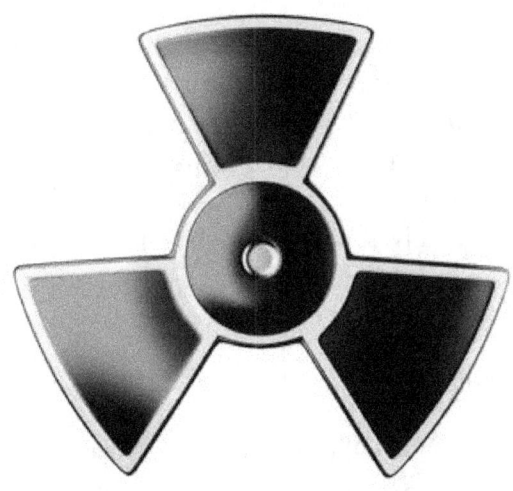

Week 1 of the Elimination phase is considered the jump week and calls for the consumption of 1 meal, an optional snack and 2 Virgin Diet shakes a day; the shakes are explained at the end of the section. The second and third weeks are called healing weeks in which you must consume 2 meals, an optional snack and 1 Virgin Diet shake; the pattern is set for a day. Throughout these weeks, make sure you note every food you eat in a health journal. The breakfast you consume must be solid yet balanced, meaning 400-500 calories; at the same time keep in mind that every food you eat must have less than 5 grams of sugar in it and always avoid eating the same foods two days in a row as they can cause imbalances in the body.

Meal schedule:

- Within an hour of waking up consume a Virgin Diet shake.

- Eat every 4-6 hours; a more ideal option for those on the diet would be consuming 2 meals followed by an afternoon snack followed by a final meal.

- Avoid eating 3 hours before bed.

Your meals should consist of:

1. **30% non-starchy vegetables**

   When consuming vegetables, it is best to eat 2 cups if eating raw or 1 cup if cooking them. Beet greens, chicory, arugula, cabbage, dandelion greens, collard greens, kale, lettuce, endive, mustard greens, spinach, turnip greens, radicchio, watercress, asparagus, artichokes, bamboo shoots, bell peppers, bean sprouts, Brussels sprouts, broccoli, cassava, celery, coriander, chives, endive, eggplant, fennel, garlic, kohlrabi, radish, parsley, onions, shallots, tomatoes and zucchini are all considered best when on this diet.

2. **25% lean proteins:**

   For women, the amount of proteins set is 4-6 ounces while for men, the amount is 6-8 ounces per meal. You may consume red meat 3 to 4 times a week, with your prime focus being on lamb and game; get the rest of the proteins from fish, chicken and Virgin shakes. Furthermore, enjoy 3 servings of low-mercury fish per week (6 oz.). butterfish, anchovies, squid, farmed caviar, catfish, king crab, clams, flounder, herring, oysters, salmon, sardines, Pollock, sole, tilapia, shrimps and whitefish. If you're a vegetarian then eat a good combination of legumes, grains, nuts, seeds and lentils.

3. **25% healthy fats:**

   A single serving of healthy fats is equal to 100 calories where you have to consume 1-3 servings per meal. 1/3 avocado, fat in grass-fed beef, lamb or cold-water fish are all eligible for consumption. Even though coconut milk, avocados, olive oil, palm fruit, and sesame oil are all great sources, the champion of healthy fats are coconut oil and red-palm fruit oil. Nuts and raw-seeds are also good sources of fats, especially if they are soaked in water overnight as this reduces the amount of dangerous chemicals in them. Ghee, milk from grass-fed cows, and clarified butter are all great sources as well.

4. **15% fiber:**

1 cup per meal for men while ½ cup for women. Legumes are great sources of fiber; legumes that could prove good in this diet are black beans, adzuki beans, chick peas, great northern beans, kidney beans lentils, mung beans, lima beans, split beans, white beans, and navy beans. Gluten free grains include brown rice, quinoa, oat bran and millet. With both types, it is best to consume soaked and fermented grains. Starchy vegetables include carrots, beets, okra, jicama, French beans, yam, pumpkins and turnip. Avoid potatoes as they have a high glycemic index.

Furthermore, consume fruits that are low to moderate in GI. Fruits with low GI include blueberries, blackberries, elderberries, boysenberries, loganberries, strawberries, gooseberries and raspberries whereas fruits with a moderate GI are oranges, grapefruit, apricots, kiwi, apples, lemons, melons, limes, cherries, nectarines, passion fruit, pear, peaches, plums, persimmons, tangerines and pomegranates. If you have a condition of insulin resistance, limit fruit intake to one per day.

The following is a list of foods that would prove most compatible to you:

i. **Proteins**: Pasture fed lamb, hormone free chicken, hemp protein, and cold water fish.

ii. **Non-starchy vegetables:** Cabbage, cauliflower, broccoli, spinach, green vegetables.

iii. **Fruits:** Blueberries, apples.

iv. **Fats:** Chia seeds, avocado, coconut milk, coconut oil, flaxseed meal, palm fruit oil.

v. **High Fiber:** Lentils, quinoa, brown rice, sweet potatoes.

Fermented foods include:

i. Pickled cabbage,

ii. Kombucha without sugar,

iii. Fermented fish,

iv. Dark chocolate,

v. Greek style yogurt.

The following is a table showing a variety of healing foods:

Apples	Avocado	Coconut milk	Artichokes
Beets	Broccoli	Curcumin	Blueberries
Cabbage	Cilantro	Olive oil	Cinnamon
Fresh garlic	Ginger	Lentils	Green tea
Palm fruit oil	Red peppers	Red onions	Sea salt
Rosemary	Sauerkraut	Seafood	Xylitol
Sweet potatoes			

Chapter 2: Reintroduction

This phase is set for 4 weeks; each week a potentially healthy food is tested and it is determined whether the food must remain a part of the diet or not; the rest of the diet remains the same as the first phase.

Week 1 – Test Soy:

Through Monday to Thursday include a meal that adds soy to your diet. From Friday to Sunday, revert back to the original diet. Trace your symptoms each day at the following website for free http://thevirgindiet.com/symptomschecklist. Continue with the consumption of at least one Virgin Diet shake every day to stay hydrated.

Week 2 – Test Gluten:

Through Monday to Thursday include a meal that carries gluten into your diet plan. The rest of the instructions are same as with Week 1.

Week 3 – Test Eggs:

Add a meal that includes eggs from Monday to Thursday and the rest is the same as Week 1.

Week 4 – Test Dairy:

From Monday to Thursday include a meal that contains dairy while the rest is the same as week 1. Note that if you can't tolerate cow's milk; include sheep's milk or goat milk. The best ways in which you can consume these types of milks are raw.

Even if you are tolerant to gluten, eggs or soy during the test period, do not add them back to the diet during the remaining weeks. If you consume a forbidden food during this time period, make sure you don't consume that food again for at least 21 days. If a response is shown on the first day then the food is not for eating; re-challenge it in 3 months. If no reaction is shown to the foods, then you may include them into your diet in the 3rd cycle.

Chapter 3: Lifetime Diet

The third cycle of the Virgin Diet is the same as cycle 1 along with the elimination of foods that you rejected in the 2nd cycle. Continue developing meals as before using the same meal proportions avoiding sugar, gluten, soy, peanuts and artificial sweeteners 95% of the time. Keep up with your cravings by using a 3-bite rule that allows you to take 3 bites of something you wouldn't normally eat, like desserts. If you had no reaction to eggs and soy, include them within your diet; if you reacted immediately, leave them for 3 months.

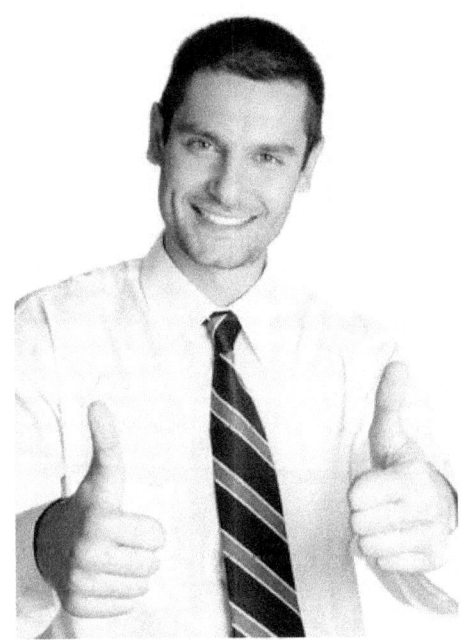

Substitute one meal each day with a Virgin shake, stay hydrated and reintroduce alcohol if you want to.

Still if you're trying to lose weight:

i.   Replace 2 meals with Virgin Diet shakes.

ii.   Replace high-fiber carbohydrates with non-starchy vegetables.

iii.   Drink more green tea.

iv.   Increase fiber intake.

v.   Stay abundantly hydrated.

vi.   Shift from high fat proteins to low fat ones; from grass-fed beef to chicken breasts.

Move through the cycles once a year for the rest of your life.

The foods that are forbidden in this diet are the same from cycle 2; furthermore reduce the consumption of alcohol to 1 glass a day for women and 2 for men.

Chapter 4: Virgin Diet Shakes

Virgin Diet Shakes are effective meal replacements aimed at providing you all the essential nutrients of a meal in a comprehensive manner. The shakes can be prepared with ease using pea-rice protein, freshly ground flaxseed, fiber, nut butter, frozen berries, and coconut milk. The recipe can be hard to master at times therefore pre-made shakes are the best choice for a beginner like you. Virgin Diet shakes can be bought in powdered form via the Amazon online store. The following are a few things you should check for when purchasing the Shakes:

- Less than 5 grams of sugar,

- No artificial sweeteners,

- No dairy, whey, eggs or soy,

- More than 5 grams fiber

- No maltodextrin

- Rice protein, hemp protein or pea protein,

- Sugar alcohols

2 scoops of the powdered shake would be enough for one shake serving.

Recipes

Chapter 1: Salmon, Arugula & Red Quinoa Salad

Makes: 4 servings

Cooking time: 20-30 minutes

Ingredients:

- 4 salmon fillets, skinless
- 1 cup white wine
- 1 sliced white onion
- ½ cup red quinoa
- 3 sprigs thyme
- ¼ cup golden raisins
- ½ cup canned chickpeas
- 1 teaspoon cinnamon, ground
- 1 teaspoon turmeric, ground
- 1 teaspoon cayenne pepper
- 1 teaspoon paprika
- Juice of 2 lemons
- 2 cups arugula
- 1 ½ tablespoons olive oil
- ½ cup cilantro leaves

- 4 tablespoons harissa

- 2 tablespoons toasted slivered almonds

Directions:

First, take a large pot and boil wine along with 4 cups of water in it. Add onion, thyme and salmon to the pot and reduce the heat so that it can simmer; poach the salmon until it is cooked; about 7 minutes. Take the salmon and allow it to cool and in a separate large pot, boil 4 cups of water; add the quinoa and cook for 11 minutes or until it turns tender. In a bowl mix the chickpeas, quinoa, spices and raisins and let them cool. Toss this mixture with arugula and dress the salad with oil and lemon juice; season with salt and pepper. Divide the poached salmon in 4 plates and top each one with 1 tablespoon harissa.

Chapter 2: Grilled Halibut with Pepper Salsa

Makes: 4 servings

Cooking time: 40 minutes

Ingredients:

- Salsa:

a. 1 cup red bell-peppers, chopped

b. 1 1/3 cups yellow peaches, peeled & coarsely chopped

c. 1/3 cup thinly sliced green onion

d. 1/4 cup lemon juice, fresh

e. 1/3 cup fresh arugula, chopped

f. 4 teaspoons fresh oregano, chopped

g. ½ habanero pepper, minced

h. 1 garlic clove, minced

- Fish:

i. 4 teaspoons lemon juice

j. ½ teaspoon paprika

k. 4 teaspoons olive oil

l. 1 garlic clove, minced

m. 3/8 teaspoon salt

n. 4 skinless halibut fillets

o. 3/8 teaspoon black pepper

p. Cooking spray

Directions:

For the salsa, combine the first 9 ingredients and let them stand for 30 minutes. Meanwhile, prepare a grill at medium heat; to prepare the fish, combine oil, paprika, lemon juice and a garlic clove in a shallow glass baking dish, stirring with a whisk. Add the fish to this mixture and properly coat it and let it stand for 15 minutes. Take the fish from the marinade; sprinkle it with 3/8 teaspoons salt and some pepper. Place the fish on a grill rack coated with spray, grilling for 3 minutes on each side. Serve the fish with salsa.

Chapter # 3: Lentil Nut Burgers

Makes: 4 servings

Cooking time: 30-40 minutes

Ingredients:

- 2 tablespoons fresh cilantro

- ½ teaspoon lime zest, grated

- 1 tablespoon lime juice

- ½ teaspoon sea salt

- 4 ounces white mushrooms

- 1 small onion, chopped

- 3 garlic cloves, minced

- 1/3 cup raw walnuts, chopped

- 1 teaspoon cumin, ground

- 1 cup brown rice

- 1 can organic lentils

- 2 tablespoons fresh parsley,

- ¼ teaspoon black pepper, freshly ground

Directions:

Combine the zest, lime juice, ¼ teaspoon salt and cilantro in a bowl, followed by 2 tablespoons of the oil in a steady stream. Set this aside and heat 2 teaspoons of the oil in a non-stick skillet over medium-high heat; add the mushrooms, garlic, cumin and onion, cooking while stirring occasionally for 5 minutes. Add the walnuts in the skillet and cook until the nuts become toasted; this would take about 3 minutes. Transfer this to a bowl and combine the rice and lentils in a food processor and pulse them so that they are coarsely chopped; add this to the mushrooms. Add in the parsley, ¼ teaspoon salt, some pepper and form four patties with ½ inch thickness. Heat 4 teaspoons oil in a skillet over medium-high heat and add these patties onto it; turning them once until they are browned; this will take about 10 minutes. Transfer the cooked product onto plates and top with cilantro vinaigrette.

Chapter # 4: Roasted Shrimp alongside Spaghetti Squash

Makes: 3 servings

Cooking time: 1 hour 30 minutes

Ingredients:

- Kosher salt & freshly ground pepper
- 1 large spaghetti squash
- 1 tablespoon + 1 teaspoon virgin olive oil
- 1 pound large shrimp
- 1 tablespoon lemon juice
- 2 tablespoons parsley

Directions:

Preheat an oven to 375 degrees Fahrenheit and season the squash using only salt and pepper. Place the cut side-down in a 9x13 baking dish and add 3/5 cups water, roasting until it turns tender; this would take about ¾ hours. After 25 minutes, toss the shrimp on a baking sheet with 1 teaspoon oil, seasoning it with salt and pepper. Roast for 10 minutes before scooping out seeds from the squash. Using a fork, scrape out the flesh into a large bowl, add shrimp, lemon juice and 1 tablespoon oil and toss so it combines thoroughly. Finally season with salt and pepper, top it up with parsley and serve alongside lemon wedges.

Chapter # 5: Tomatillo & Black Bean Soup

Makes: 4 servings

Cooking time: 40 – 50 minutes

Ingredients:

- 2 red onions
- 12 small tomatillos
- 2 jalapeno peppers
- Olive oil
- 3 garlic cloves
- Kosher salt
- 1 can beans
- 1 can hominy
- 1 quart vegetable broth
- 2 sprigs cilantro
- 8 radishes
- 3 green onions
- Freshly ground pepper
- Lime

Directions:

First, preheat an oven to 450 degrees Fahrenheit; roughly chop the 12 small tomatillos, 2 jalapeno peppers and 2 red onions and cut the garlic cloves into quarters. Place the chopped veggies and garlic onto a baking sheet lined with parchment paper and drizzle with oil enough to coat it. Sprinkle with kosher salt and roast until the veggies are softly browned. Meanwhile, rinse the black beans and hominy plus prepare thin slices of onions and radishes to be used as garnishes. Add the roasted veggies to a pot and use an immersion blender to puree with a quart of vegetable broth. Add 3 sprigs of cilantro, black beans and hominy, bringing the mixture to a boil followed by lowering of the heat for 15 minutes. Remove the cilantro sprigs and pour into bowls; garnish as per desire.

Chapter # 6: Sweet Potato Black Bean Burger

Makes: 8 burgers

Cooking time: 1 hour and 30 minutes

Ingredients:

- Burger:

i. ½ cup dry millet

ii. ½ cup rolled oats

iii. 1 medium sweet potato

iv. 2 tablespoons fresh cilantro

v. 1 ½ teaspoons garlic powder

vi. ½ teaspoon salt

vii. 1 teaspoon cumin

viii. ½ teaspoon pepper

ix. 1 cup corn

x. 15 ounce black beans

xi. 2 tablespoons olive oil

xii. 8 whole-wheat burger buns

- Cream sauce:

i. 3 ounces nonfat Greek yogurt

ii. 1 teaspoon fresh lime juice

iii. 1 ripe avocado

iv.   1 Roma tomato

v.   ¼ teaspoon salt

Directions:

Preheat an oven to 400 degrees Fahrenheit and bake the sweet potato for 60 minutes. While the potato is baking, cook the millet for 30 minutes; cool the baked potato and combine it with oats, black beans, garlic powder, cilantro, salt and pepper, cumin and a tablespoon of oil in a food processor. Mix well until smooth. Then, in a separate bowl, mix the potato mixture with millet, beans and corn. Heat the remaining oil in a large pan and place spoonfuls of the mixture onto the pan. Use the back of the spoon to form 4 inch thick patties and cook until both sides of the burger are browned. In the meantime, mash the avocado using a fork and add in the yogurt, lime juice, salt and tomatoes. Serve the patties on a bun with a dollop of the cream sauce.

Chapter # 7: Roasted Brussels sprouts Chips

Makes: 4 servings

Cooking time: 30 minutes

Ingredients:

- 10 Brussels sprouts

- ¼ teaspoon kosher salt

- 1 tablespoon olive oil

Directions:

Preheat an oven to 350 degrees Fahrenheit. Using a paring knife, cut the bottom part of each sprout so that the tiny leaves fall off; continue to do so until all the leaves have been removed. Toss the leaves into oil and lay them in rimmed baking sheet afterwards, roasting for 10 minutes until they turn crispy.

Chapter # 8: Protein-Packed Salad

Makes: 4 servings

Cooking time: 10 minutes

Ingredients:

- 1 cup cooked quinoa

- 3 cups cooked beans

- 1 deseeded sweet, red pepper

- 1 big parsley

- 1 leek

- 2 carrots

And for the dressing:

i.   1 teaspoon chili oil

ii.   2 tablespoon olive oil

iii.   2 tablespoon cider vinegar

iv.   1 clove garlic

v.   Some balsamic vinegar

vi.   Salt & pepper to taste

Directions:

Chop the peppers, leeks, parsley and carrots and combine them with beans and quinoa in a large bowl. Mix the dressing ingredients, thoroughly and add them to the salad. Give the salad a final mix and serve.

Conclusion

The book offers a comprehensive guidance to the Virgin Diet and ways to successfully implement it in one's life. The work of JJ Virgin has proved ground breaking and unlike other diets, and actually does provide the best bang for your buck. The diet itself is not a tedious one and even a slightly motivated individual can reap its benefits. The warnings, the cycles and the recipes, all have been provided in this book so that you can best make it a coherent part of your life.

Now, the ball's in your court; either follow it and lose weight, the intelligent way or continue to be a testing ground for more Diet plans that just won't work.

Best of luck!

References

http://www.fotolia.com/id/42606253

http://www.fotolia.com/id/45319152

http://www.fotolia.com/id/45257208

http://www.fotolia.com/id/52133132

http://www.fotolia.com/id/51102457

http://www.fotolia.com/id/56739227

http://www.123rf.com/photo_11272267_soy-milk-with-beans-in-spoon.html

Author Bio

Muhammad Usman is a distinguished medical graduate of Allama Iqbal medical college (AIMC). He is a professional writer who has been in the field for more than 4 years. During this time he has produced 10,000+ articles, blogs and eBooks on various niches related to diseases, health, fitness, nutrition and well-being. He is a regular contributor to several journals related to medicine and surgery. He is the editor of several journals and newspapers.

Check out some of the other JD-Biz Publishing books

Gardening Series on Amazon

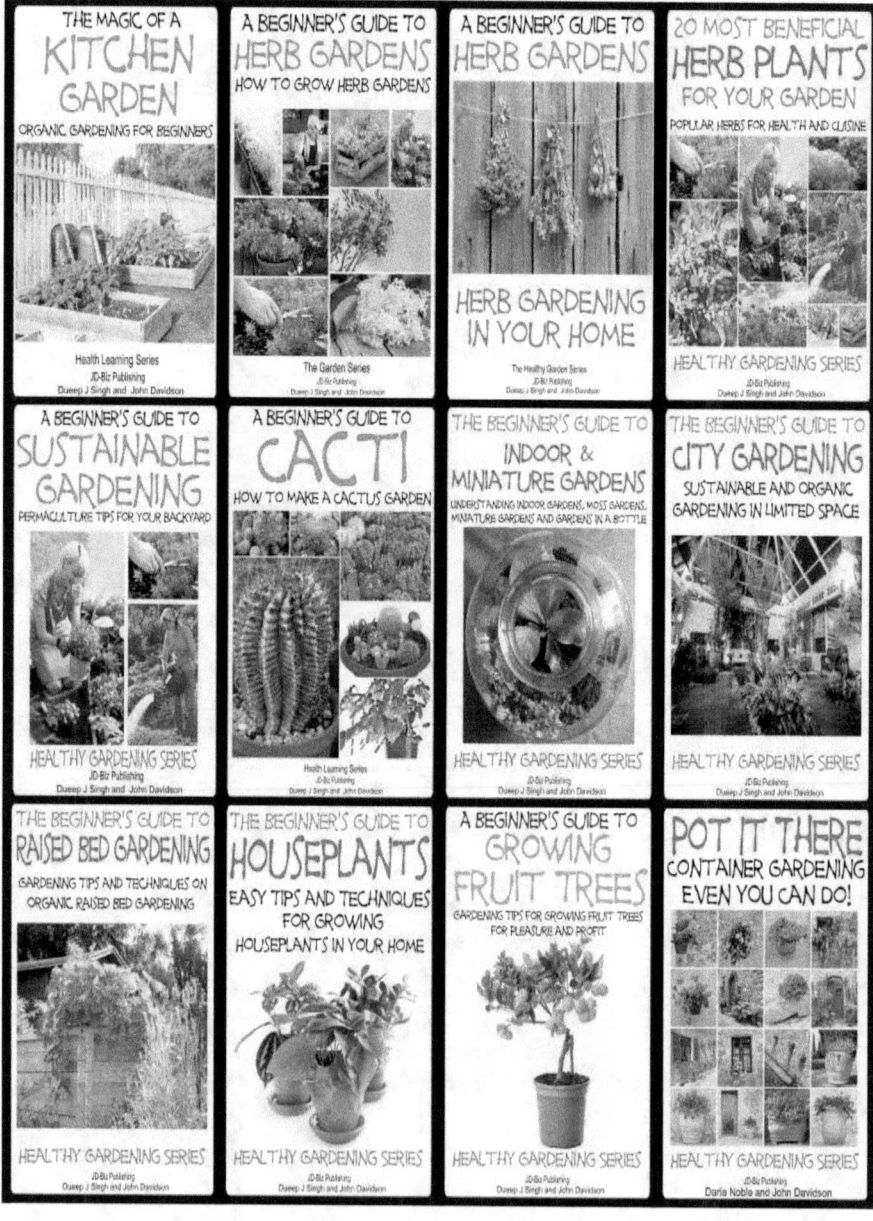

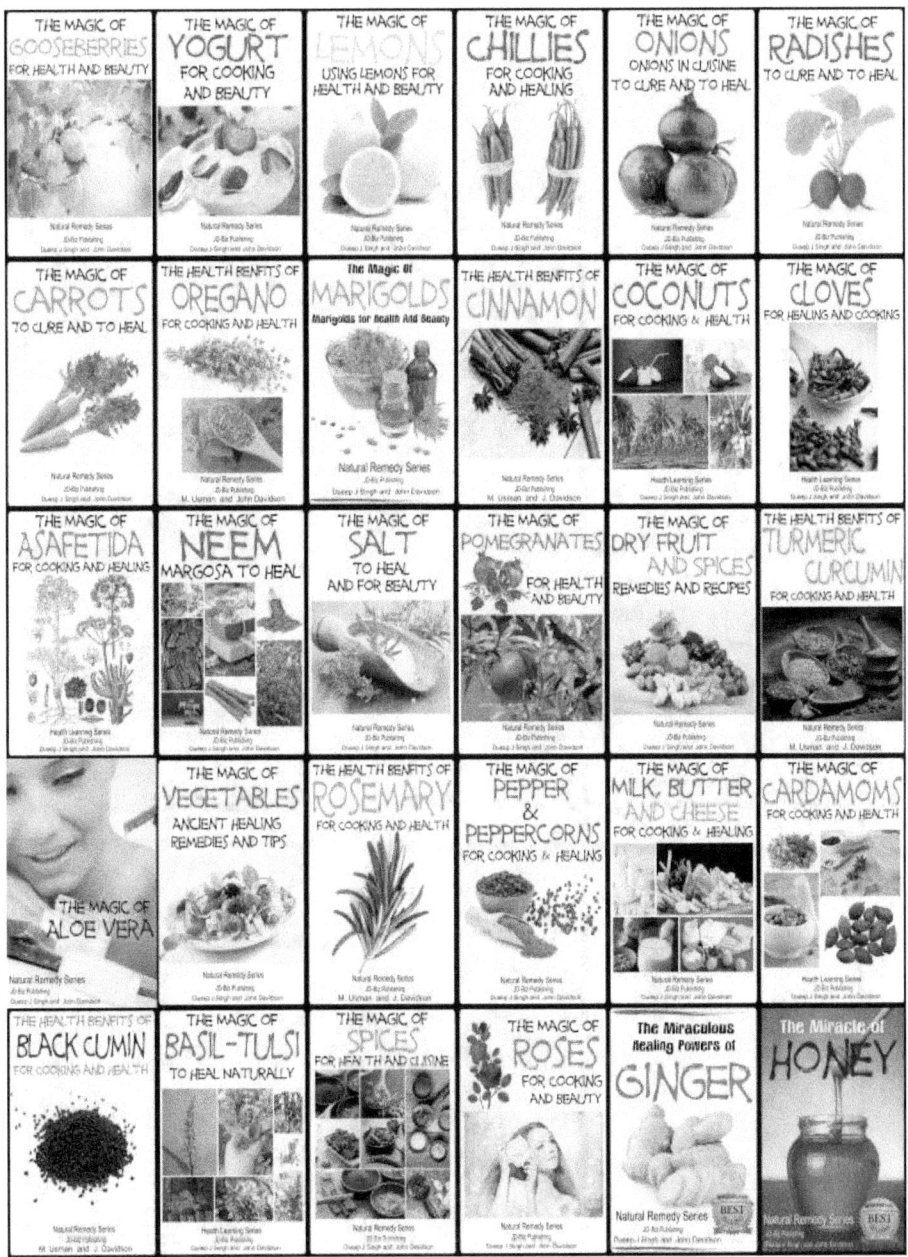

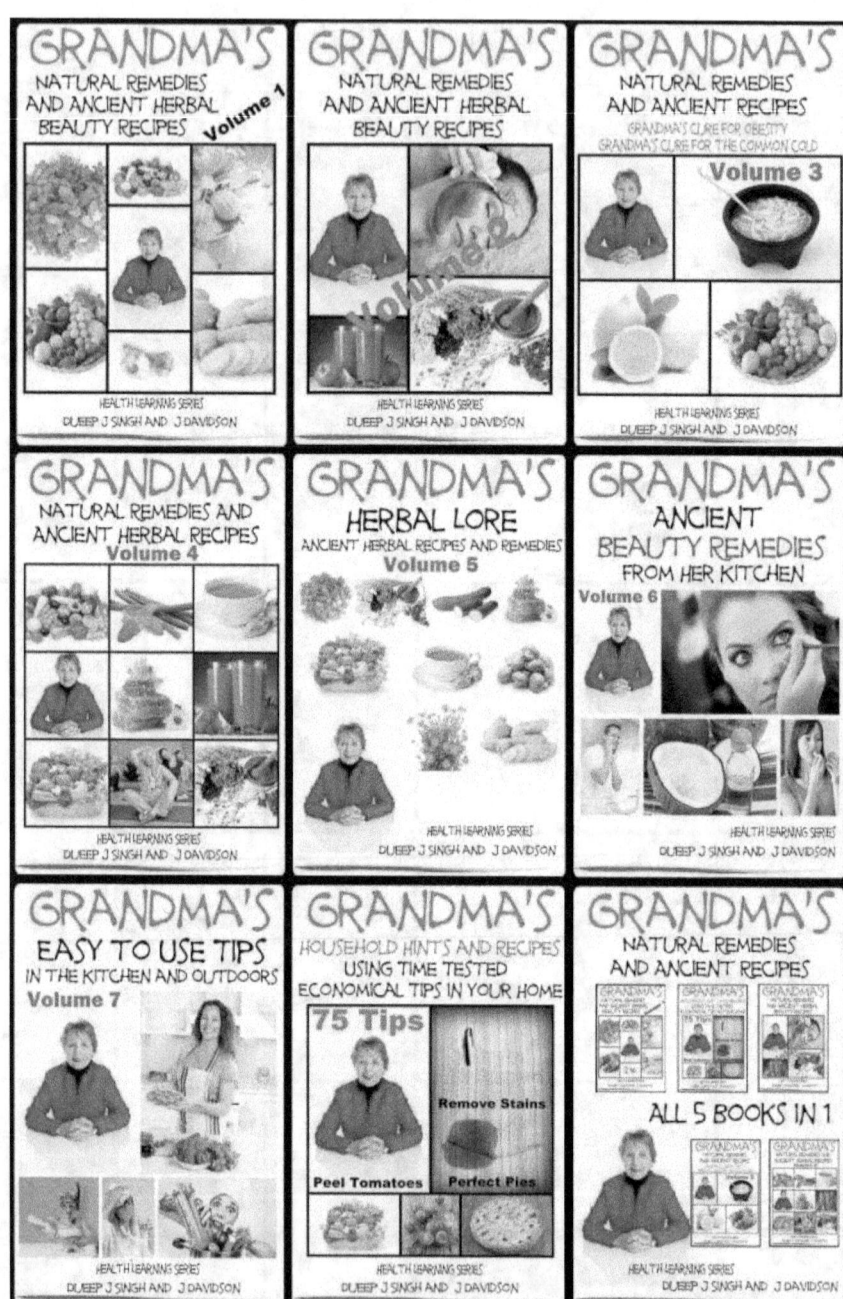

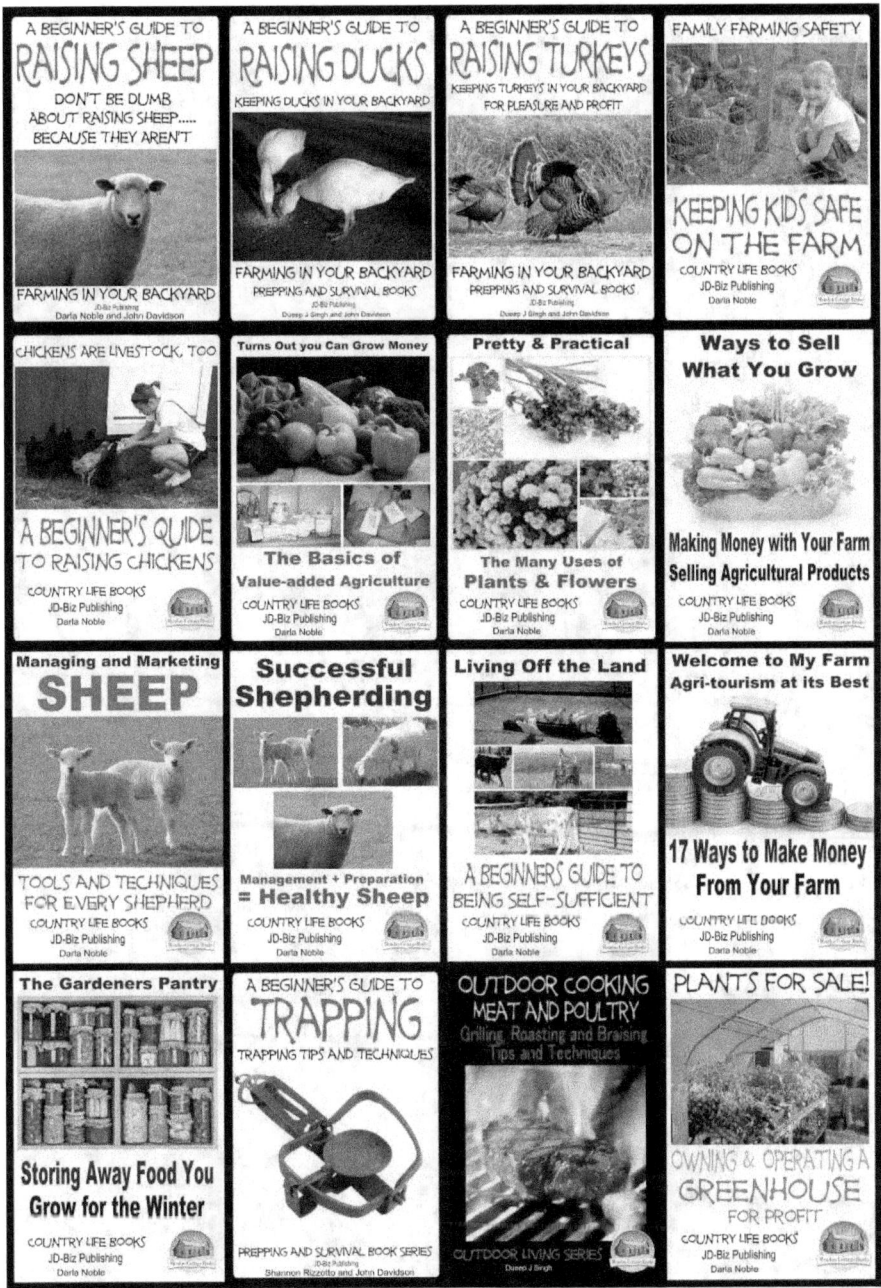

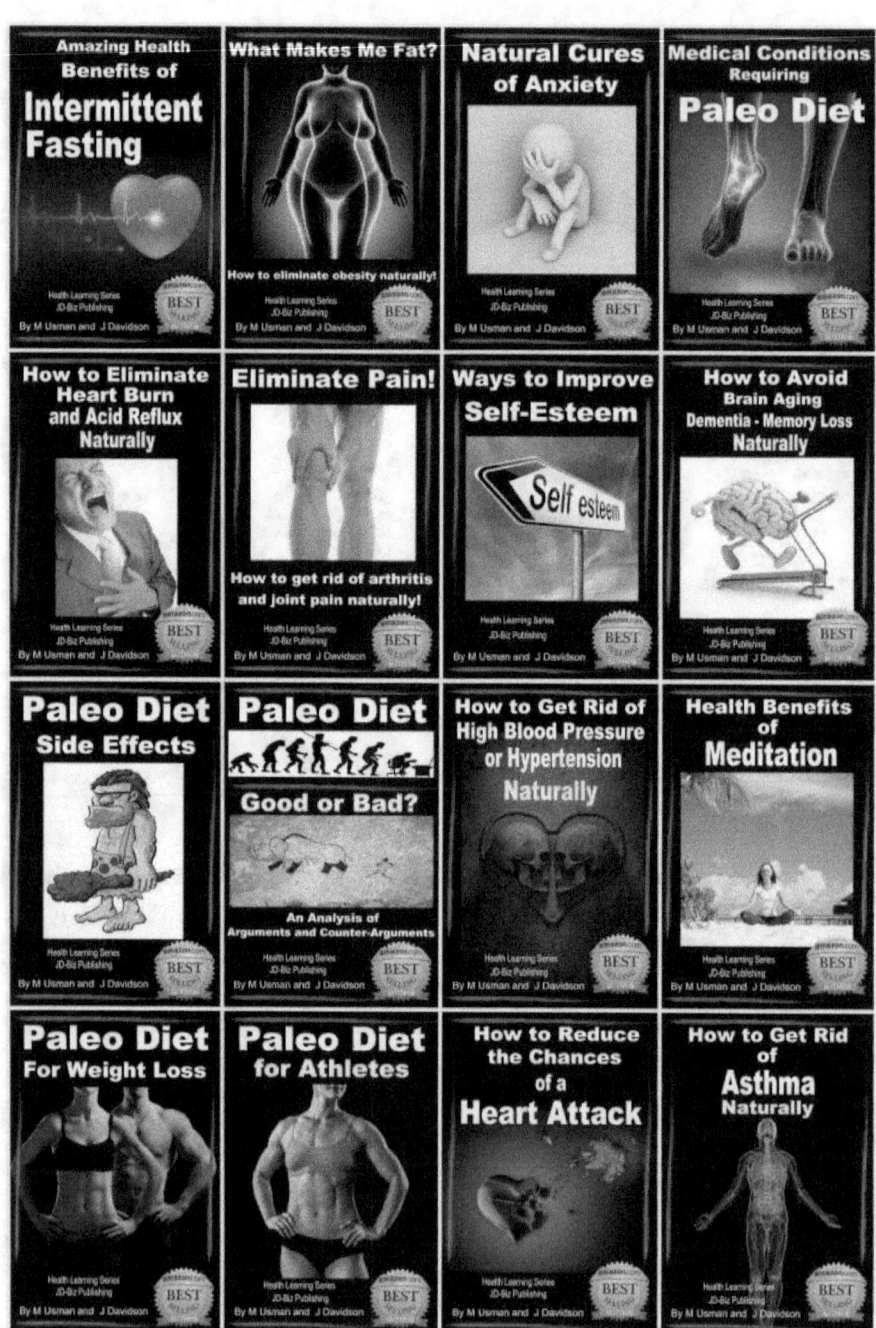

Amazing Animal Book Series

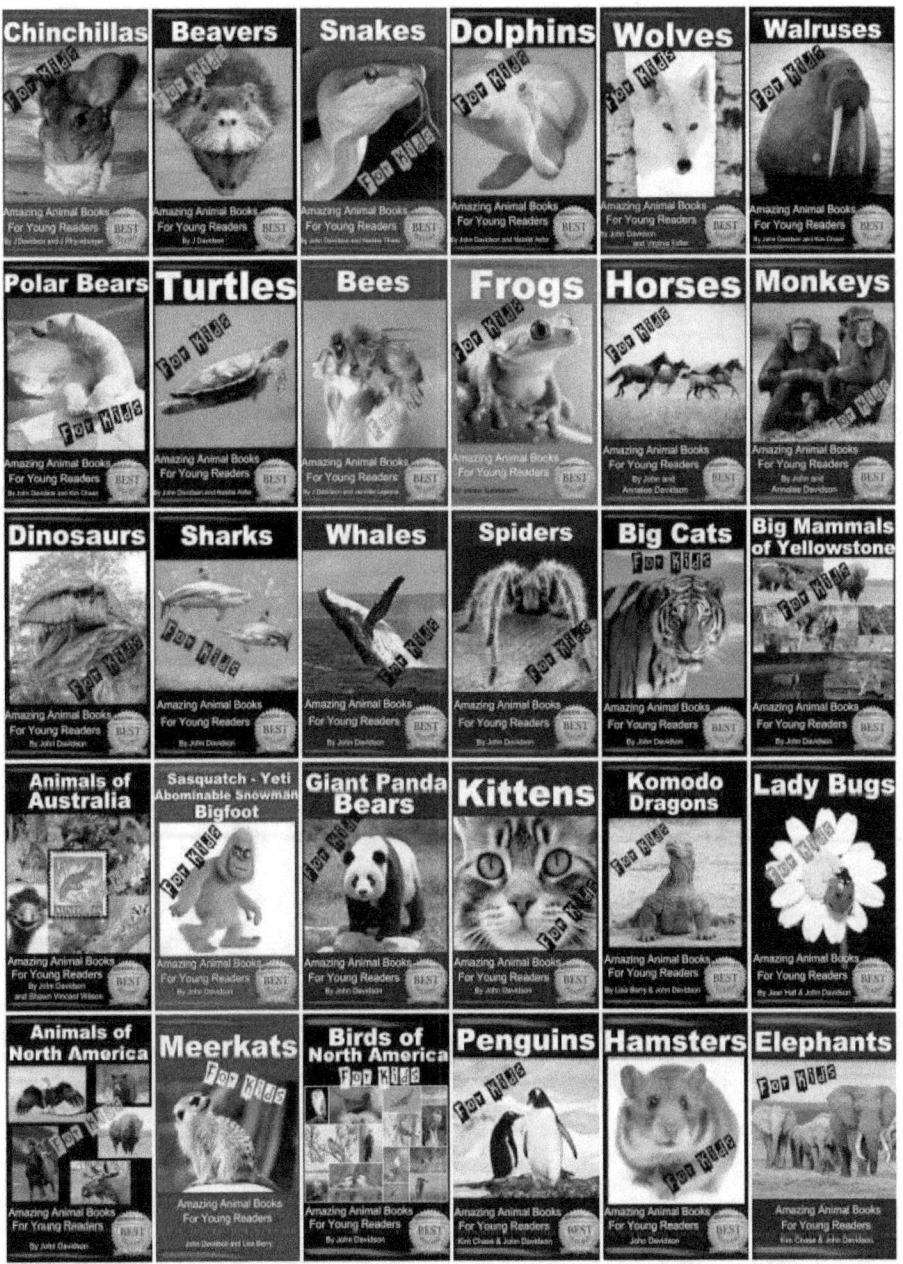

Learn To Draw Series

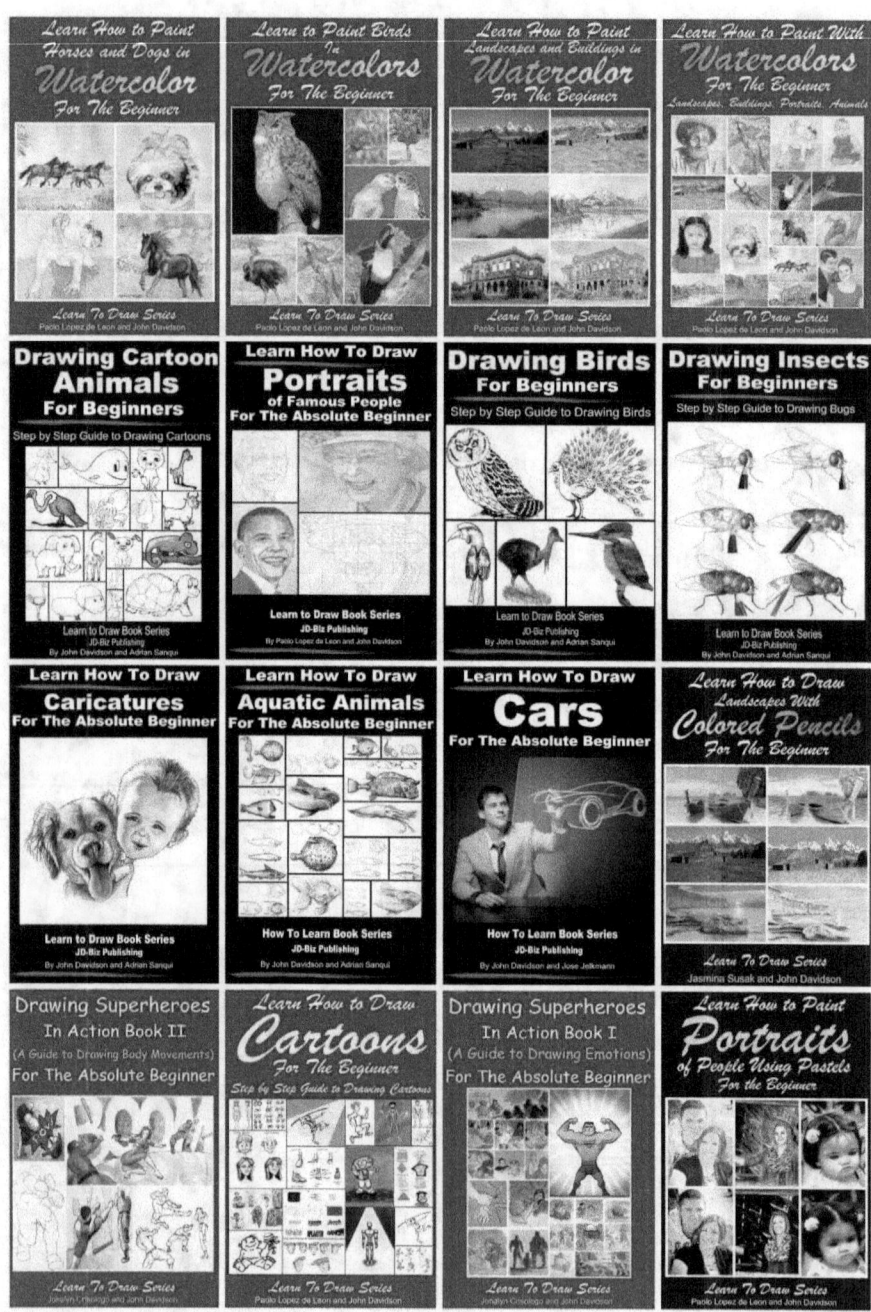

How to Build and Plan Books

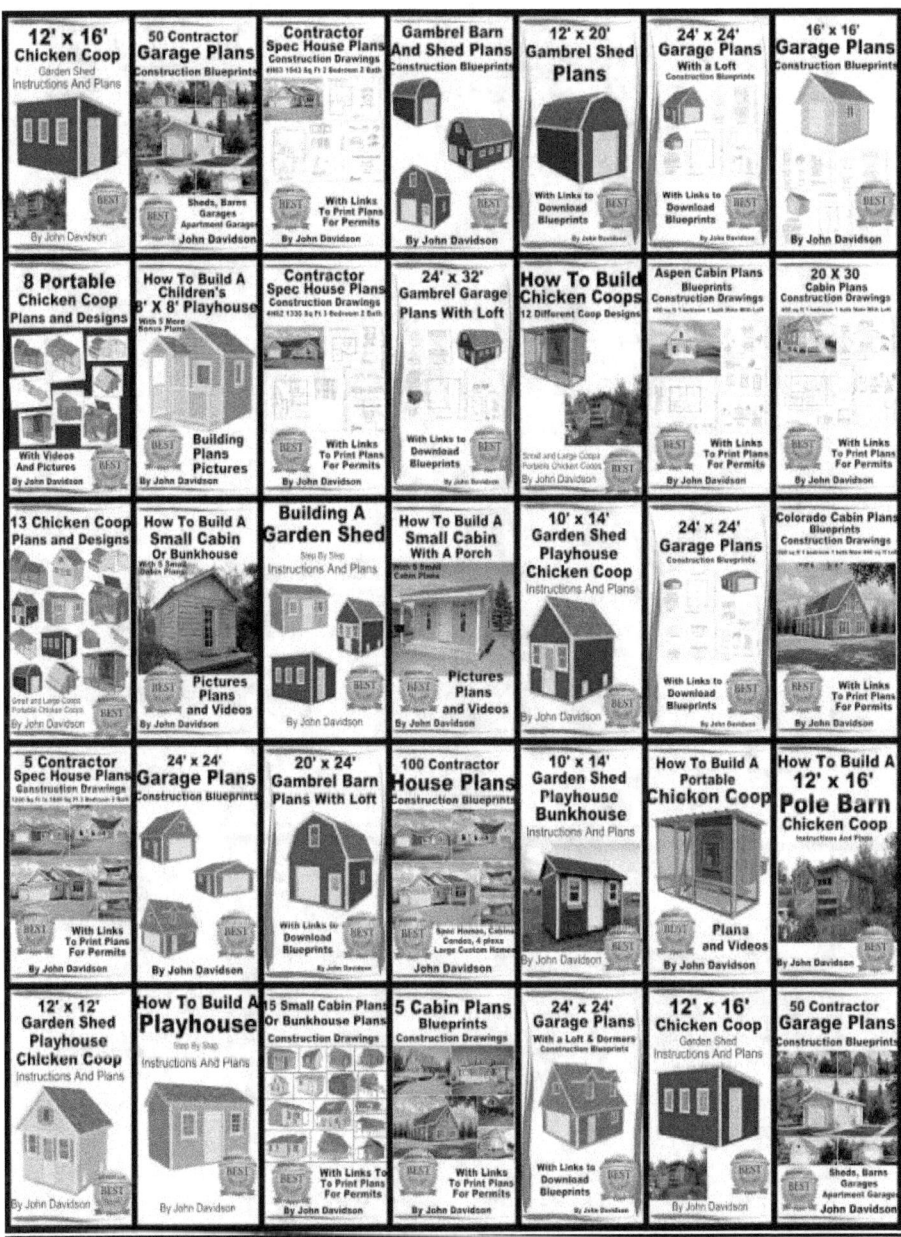

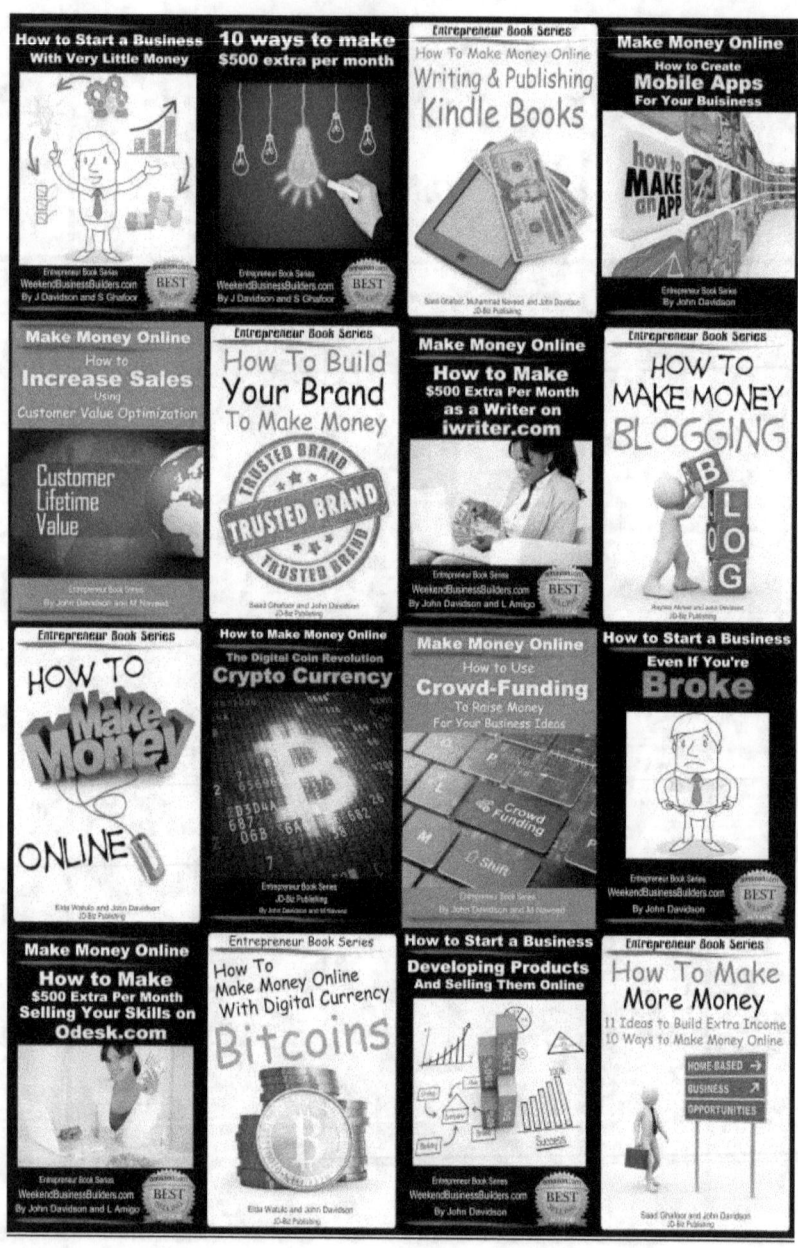

Our books are available at

1. Amazon.com

2. Barnes and Noble

3. Itunes

4. Kobo

5. Smashwords

6. Google Play Books

Publisher

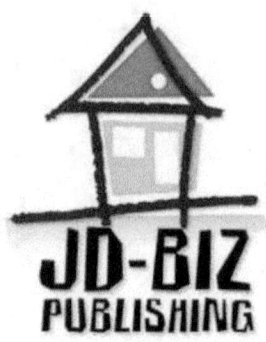

JD-Biz Corp

P O Box 374

Mendon, Utah 84325

http://www.jd-biz.com/

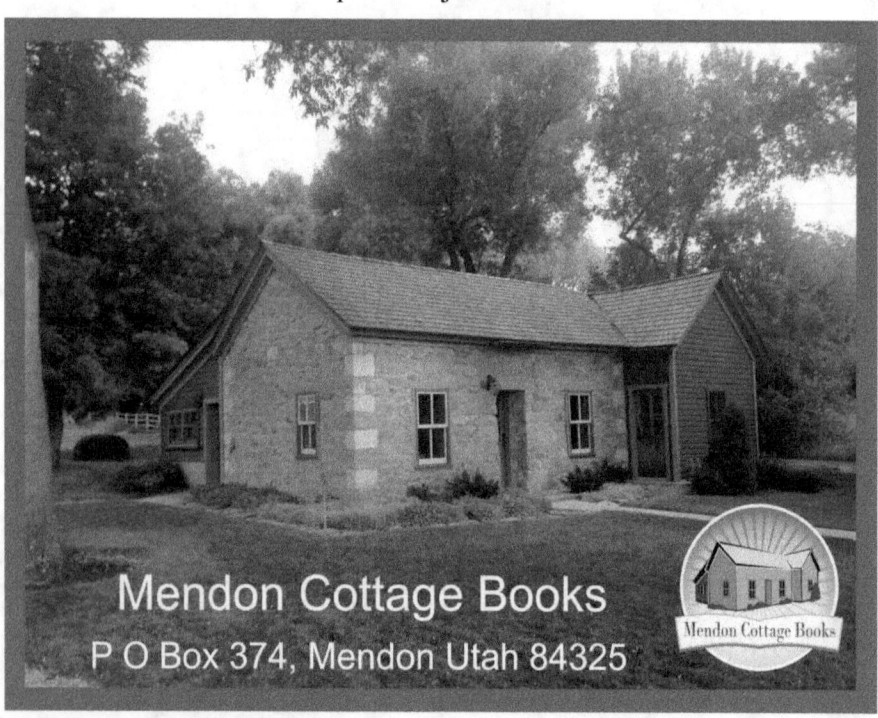

Mendon Cottage Books

P O Box 374, Mendon Utah 84325